CANDLE LIGHT DINNER: TOXIC RIDDLE FOR THE TOXIC DETECTIVE

An Indian Society of Toxicology Initiative

Dr Vivekanshu Verma
Dr Vijay Vasudev Pillay
Dr Shiv Rattan Kochar
Dr Prateek Rastogi
Dr. Shweta H Patel

Indian Society of Toxicology
Poison Control Centre
Amrita Institute of Medical Science,
Ponekkara, P. O, Kochi, Kerala - 682041.

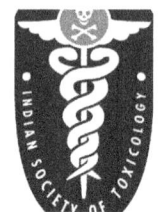

Copyright © 2020 © Indian Society of Toxicology

All rights reserved

The characters and events portrayed in this book are fictitious.
Any similarity to real persons, living or dead, is coincidental and not intended by the author.

No part of this book may be reproduced, or stored in a retrieval system, or transmitted in any form or by any means, electronic, mechanical, photocopying, recording, or otherwise, without express written permission of the publisher.

ISBN:9798588795739

Cover design by: Vishwendra verma
Library of Indian Society of Toxicology Archive Number: 2018675309
Printed in the Poison Control Centre
Amrita Institute of Medical Science,
Ponekkara, P. O, Kochi, Kerala - 682041.

DR VIVEKANSHU VERMA FIST

Candle Light Dinner: Toxic Riddle for the Toxic Detective

An Indian Society of Toxicology Initiative

For Toxic Detectives, Crime Scene Investigators (CSi), Toxicologists, Police Officers, CID & CBI officers, Lawyers, Judges, Magistrates, Legal counsels, Law Students, Forensic Scientists, Doctors, Toxicology Nurses & Emergency Paramedics

Dr Vivekanshu Verma, MBBS, Postgraduate Diploma in Forensic Medicine & Toxicology, Fellow of Indian Society of Toxicology, Associate consultant, Emergency & Trauma care, Medanta-The Medicity, Gurugram. Honorary Toxicology Expert, Central Bureau of Investigation

Dr Vijay Vasudev Pillay, MBBS, MD Forensic Medicine & Toxicology, Chief, Poison Control Centre, Professor & Head, Forensic Medicine & Toxicology, Amrita School of Medicine, Amrita Vishwa Vidyapeetham, Cochin, Kerala

Dr Shiv Rattan Kochar, MBBS, MD Forensic Medicine & Toxicology, Senior Professor, Forensic Medicine. Chief Vigilance Officer, Metro MANAS Arogya Sadan Heart Care & Multispecialty Hospital, Directorate of Medical Education, Jaipur (Rajasthan)

Dr Prateek Rastogi, MBBS,MD, PGDMLE, PGDCFS, PGCMNCPA, PGCTM, Dip. Cyber Law, FAGE, FAIMER Fellow (MUFILIPE-Manipal), Former President, Indian Society of Toxicology(2018-19), Professor, Department of Forensic Medicine & Toxicology, Kasturba Medical College, Mangalore, Karnataka.

Dr. Shweta H Patel, MBBS, MD Forensic Medicine & Toxicology, Assistant Professor, Forensic Medicine & Toxicology, Pramukhswami Medical College, Karamsad. Dist. Anand, Gujarat.

ISBN: 9798588795739

©2020 Indian Society of Toxicology

Poison Control Centre

Amrita Institute of Medical Science,

Ponekkara, P. O, Kochi, Kerala - 682041.

202ND TOXIC RIDDLE IN RHYMES

While U enjoy New Year 5 Candle light dinner & joke
Do you know, hell oil was used to make candle wax
Pin on, oil soften hard faeces remove ♠ rectum choke
As physician nuts employ, made rectal sphincter lax
Ornamental shrub, grows 5 feet tall in wild bloke;
I relieve hurting Bellyache, Bush thus make U relax
5 petal cure queue some AC cool to wind broke;
Palmate 5 lobes, like 5 Fingers in Ur Hands ▢ seen
My beans look-alike beetles blackened with 5 -spoke;
In past folk-remedies for aborting illegally in teen;
Grown industrial biodiesel use in landscaping cloak;
So cherries removed by farmers, before mature in,
Oil-rich seed$5 toxicity known to by seizure & choke,
5 Leaves have serrated margins as the weed, been
Barb 'A' dose nuts in triple-seed capsule to convoke
Use to make pesticides, varnishes, synthetic resins
As Nettle spurges, use 5 PPE Equipments, folks
Gloves, Mask ,Gown Shoes Goggles shields
Oil in poison nut & ripe fruit, yellow alike egg yolks

So i'm used as ⚡Live fences to guard grain fields
Toxic to sicken animals trespass 5 seeds to☐ poke
Diterpenoids of four ball ☠carcinogenic into yields
I'm experimental hemostatic agent, if bleed soaks
In lower concentrate, i'm anticoagulant cure stroke
Genetic engineer, non-toxic variety cultured seeds
Multipurpose herbal goldmine, enrich bean soaks
My stem bark latex is used to hunt fishing to needs
Vomiting, delirium, diarrhea symptoms, U spoke
As atropine used, relieves to Jay atropine leads
Atropine like toxidrome reported ➤ in multifida broke
I do cause black vomit nut if the victim animal feeds

CANDLE LIGHT DINNER: TOXIC RIDDLE FOR THE TOXIC DETECTIVE

2️⃣0️⃣2️⃣nd 🔍 Toxic Riddle in 💎 Rhymes
While U enjoy 🎉 New Year 5️⃣ Candle 🕯 light dinner & joke
Do you know, 🏚 hell oil was used to make candle 🕯 wax
Pin on, 🕯 oil soften hard faeces remove ⚰ rectum choke
As 👨‍⚕️ physician nuts employ, made rectal sphincter 😌 lax
Ornamental 🌿 shrub, grows 5️⃣ feet 📏 tall in wild bloke;
I relieve hurting 😣 Bellyache, Bush thus make U relax
5️⃣ petal 🌸 🌱 cure queue some AC cool to wind broke;
Palmate 🍃 5️⃣ lobes, like 5️⃣ Fingers in Ur Hands ✋ seen
My beans look-alike beetles blackened with 5️⃣-spoke;
In past 👵 folk-remedies for aborting 🤰 illegally in teen;
Grown industrial 🏭 biodiesel use in landscaping cloak;
So 🤢 cherries removed by 👨‍🌾 farmers, before mature in,
Oil-rich seeds 5️⃣ toxicity known to ⚕ by seizure & choke,
5️⃣ Leaves 🍁 have serrated margins as the 🌾 weed, been
Barb 'A' dose nuts in 🟤 triple-seed capsule 🗡 to convoke
Use to make 🧪 pesticides, varnishes, synthetic 🟥 resins
As Nettle 🌿 spurges, use 5️⃣ PPE Equipments, 👕 folks
Gloves, Mask 😷 ,Gown 👘 Shoes 👞 Goggles👓 shields
Oil in poison 😵 nut & ripe fruit, yellow alike egg 🥚 yolks
So i'm 🚩 used as ⚡ Live fences 🦗 to guard grain fields
Toxic to sicken 🐕 animals trespass 5️⃣ seeds to 🌿 poke
Diterpenoids 🌿 of four 🏀 ball ☠ carcinogenic into yields
I'm experimental 😌 hemostatic agent, if bleed 🩸 soaks
In lower 🐶 concentrate, i'm 🧠 anticoagulant cure stroke
Genetic 🧬 engineer, non-toxic variety cultured 🌱 seeds
Multipurpose 🧖 herbal goldmine, enrich 😌 bean soaks
My stem 🌿 bark latex is used to hunt 🎣 fishing to needs
Vomiting, 😵 delirium, diarrhea 😷 symptoms, U spoke
As 😵 atropine used, relieves 😀 to Jay 🐦 atropine leads
🤢 Atropine like toxidrome reported 📝 in multifida broke
I do cause 🤮 black vomit 🥜 nut if the victim animal feeds

5'S FOR EASY RECALL

All 5's Mnemonic:-

- 5 uses of Jatropha: pesticide, candle wax, biodiesel oil, Resin, varnish.
- One of the 5 most common poisonous weeds in India: Dhatura (Atropha), Jatropha, Castor, Oleander, Calotropis.
- Jatropha Shrub (Height 5 feet);
- Jatropha Tree (Height 5 meters);
- Leaves: dark green; alternate, simple, ovate to slightly lobed with 3-5 indentations.
- Leaves Up to 5 inch wide.
- Petioles 4-5 inches) long.
- Palmate Leaves are 5 lobed, alike a palm with 5 fingers;
- Flowers have 5 petals;
- Flowers: yellow to green in colour, borne in axils of the leaves and being small are mostly hidden by foliage.
- Fruit: small capsule-like, round fruit; about 2.5 - 5 cm in diameter (egg sized).
- 5-6 fruits in a bunch on branch;
- Fruit Seeds capsule: 20 mm long, has 5-6 spokes on its capsule, when dried.
- Fatal Dose: 5-6 seeds consumed by one adult human causes toxicity
- 5-Routes- Intranasal, Inhalational, oral, Intravenous, Intramuscular beneath
- 5 toxins; Phorbol, curcusone A & C, curcin or jatrophin, Curcanoleic acid & Tetramethylpyrazine.
- Curcin in endosperm of jatropha can inactivate >500

ribosomes beneath, leading to cytotoxic inhibition of protein synthesis, necrosis and cell death (apoptosis).
- For the adult male rats, the LD50 values were >500mg/kg (IP, slightly toxic) >5000 mg/kg (oral, slightly toxic)
- cause fatal 5-symptoms of irritation to vital organs perceived;

➢ Irritation to GIT- Diarrhea, Vomiting, Black vomitus, dehydration, when in feed;

➢ Corrosion to GIT- hematemesis, melena, Hypovolemia;

➢ Irritation to Respiratory tract-dyspnoea, cough & Bleeding deemed;

➢ Irritate victim's Brain- causing seizure, fits & hypoxic damage indeed;

➢ Irritate victim's Heart- arrhythmia, Hypotension, heart failure proceed;

- Within <5 hours, toxic effects to 5-organs- Brain, Adrenals, kidneys, liver, heart diseased;
- Labs show 5-abnormals:- leukocytosis, electrolyte abnormalities, liver failure, renal failure, and coagulopathy increased;
- 5 PPE equipment: Gloves, mask, cap, goggles to protect healthcare worker from secondary exposure
- For oral exposures, activated charcoal● of 50gm (another five) be given within 50-60min, in heed.
- Average recovery time is 5 – 6 hours of oral ingestion, after correcting dehydration due to diarrhoea, by intravenous fluids or ORS (Oral Rehydration Solution)

HIGH RISK GEOGRAPHICAL AREAS

Found in tropical countries throughout the world; including tropical America, warmer parts of Australia (Queensland and the Northern Territory), Florida (chiefly south of Orlando), Hawaiian Islands and Africa (Mozambique, Zambia, Transvaal, Natal), Asia (India, Indonesia).

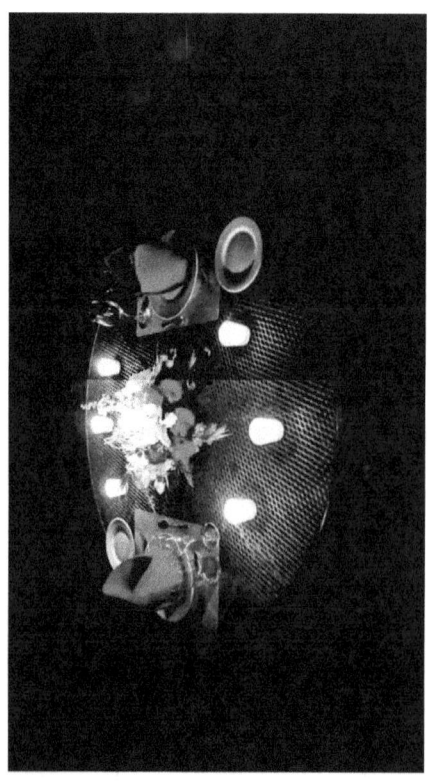

WHILE YOU ENJOY NEW YEAR IN 5 CANDLE LIGHT DINNER & JOKE

5 candle lights illuminate the entire dinner table, but in our riddle, it reminds of all 5's mnemonic for recalling the unique features of toxic plant from which candle wax is prepared.

Joke tagline:

There's nothing more romantic than the candle lights, which hides the dirty dishes & utensils.

DR VIVEKANSHU VERMA FIST

love is...

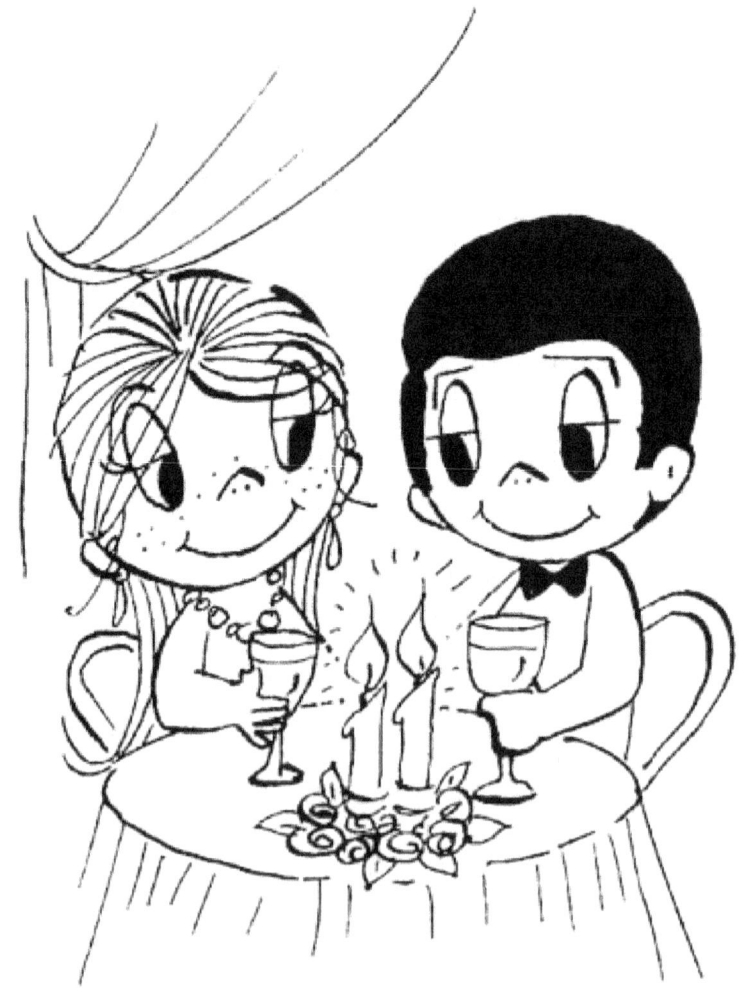

NAME:

Ratna-jyot, as its oil was a popular fuel to burn lamps in past, when electric bulb was not invented.

Jyot in Hindi means to enlighten.

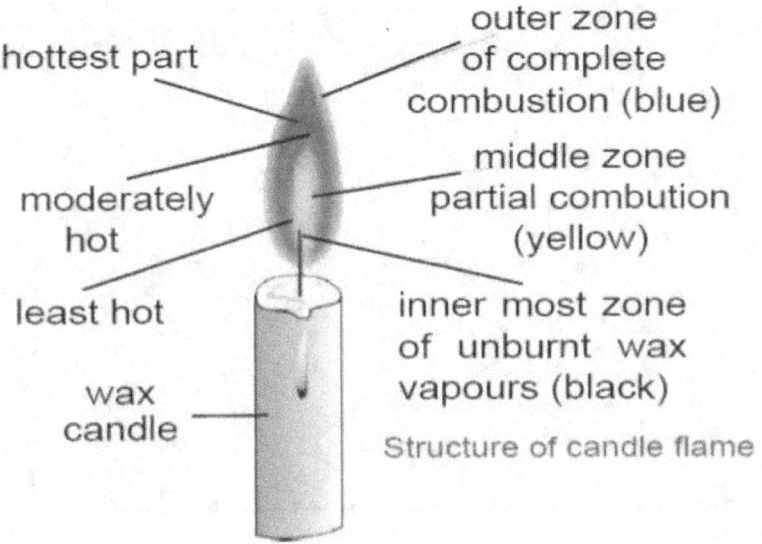

Structure of candle flame

Its seed is size of a black gem (aka Ratna in hindi) = 20 mm long.

So the sanskrit name Ratna-jyot, explains its popular use to enlighten candles like gems.

DR VIVEKANSHU VERMA FIST

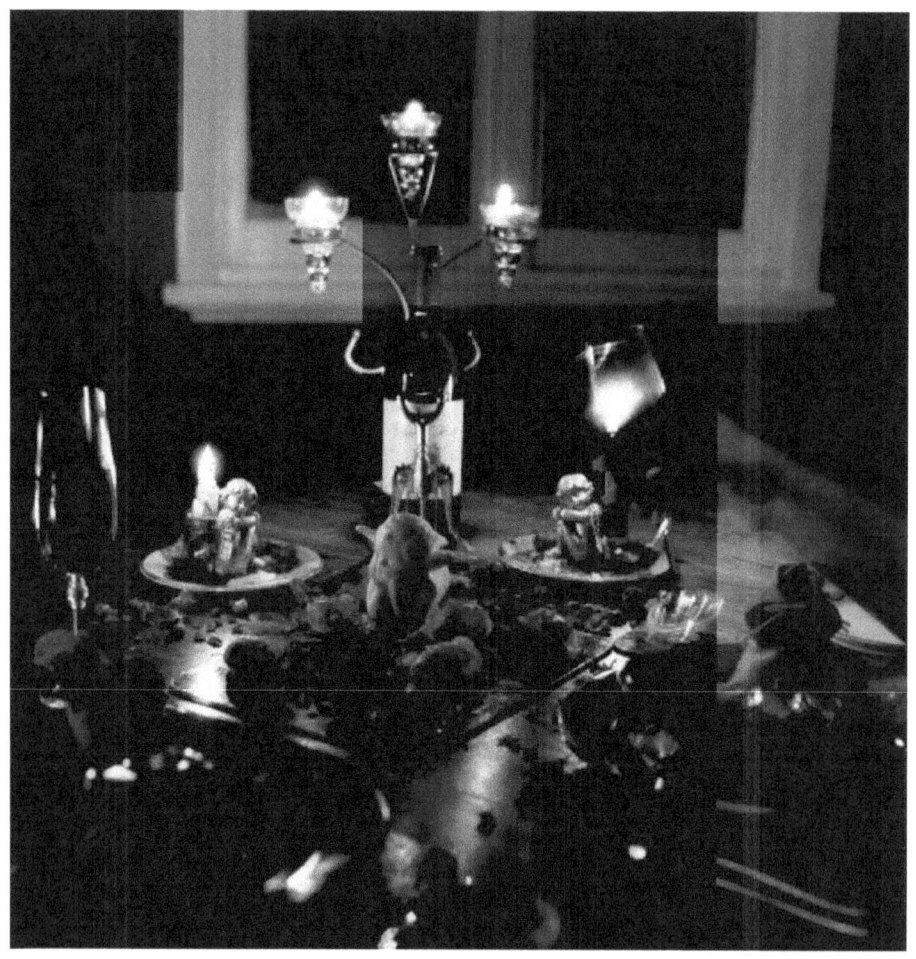

DO YOU KNOW, MY SEEDS WERE USED TO MAKE CANDLE WAX

Over the centuries, candle waxes have been developed from a variety of fats, oils and waxy-like substances derived from animals, insects, plants and rocks.

Scientists consider "wax" to be a generic term for classifying materials that have the following characteristics:

- Solid at room temperature; liquid at higher temperatures
- Primarily hydrocarbon in structure
- Water repellent; insoluble in water
- Smooth texture; buffable under slight pressure
- Low toxicity; low reactivity
- Low odor

Waxes are widely used throughout the world for a range of applications, including packaging, coatings, cosmetics, foods, adhesives, inks, castings, crayons, chewing gum, polishes and – of course – candles.

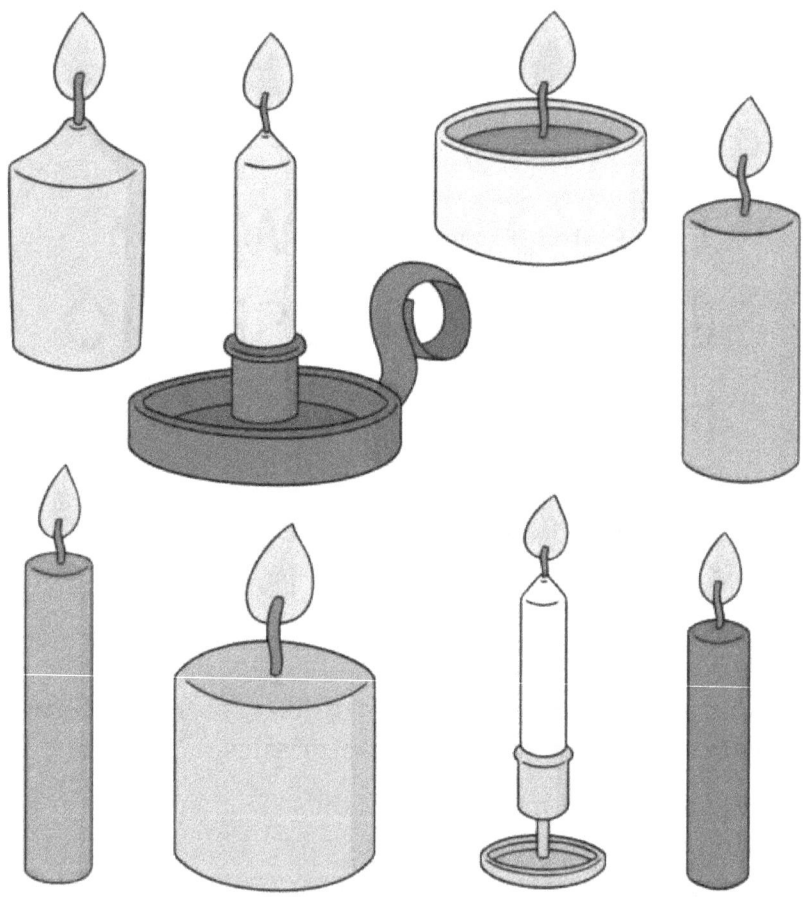

Early civilizations depended largely on the raw materials at hand to create candle wax. Ancient Egyptians and the Early Romans relied largely on tallow rendered from animals.

"A tallow candle, to be good, must be half Sheep's Tallow and half Cow's; that of hoggs mekes 'em gutter, give an ill smell, and a thick black smoak"

– Anonymous, 18th Century

In China, beeswax was used for candles as early as the Tang Dynasty (618-907 A.D.), and candle wax derived from the Coccos pella insect had been developed by the 12th century. Extracts from tree nuts were used to make candle wax in early Japan, while in India they boiled the fruit of the cinnamon tree for candle wax.

Beeswax was introduced to Europe in the Middle Ages, but was rarely used in homes because of its great expense.

Over the centuries, the development of new waxes for candles has hinged on the availability of the raw material, the ease and economy of processing the raw material into a wax suitable for candle use, and the desirability of the wax in comparison to other available candle waxes.

Tallow was the typical everyday candle wax used in Europe and the Americas until the 18th century, when the whaling industry stimulated the development of spermaceti wax, a clean-burning, low-odor wax derived from the head oil of the sperm whale.

Spermaceti remained the primary candle wax until the mid-1800s, when stearin wax and then paraffin wax were developed.

Stearin wax, based on extracting stearic acid from animal fatty acids, was widely used in Europe.

Paraffin wax, developed after chemists found a way to remove the naturally-occurring waxy substance from petroleum during refining, became the standard candle wax in the Western Hemisphere.

During the latter half of the 20th century, several synthetic and chemically synthesized waxes, including gels, were developed largely for specialty candle uses.

Two vegetable-based candle waxes – soy wax and palm wax –

were developed for commercial use in the candle market during the late 1990s by hydrogenating soybean and palm oils, respectively.

Paraffin is by far the most frequently used candle wax on a worldwide basis today.

Beeswax is also used around the globe, although in significantly smaller quantities.

Stearin candle wax is largely limited to European use.

Soy wax, palm wax, gels, synthetic waxes, and synthesized waxes are also now used in candles, as are a variety of wax blends and customized wax formulations.

MY OIL SOFTEN HARD FAECES REMOVE THE RECTUM CHOKE,

Planned Candle light dinners get spoiled, if anyone of the two in couple, is suffering from bellyache of constipation.

JATROPHA FROM IATRO-TROPHE

The name Jatropha is derived from the Greek words ἰατρός (iatros), meaning "physician," and τροφή (trophe), meaning "nutrition" and are used in traditional folklore medicine to cure various ailments in Africa, Asia and Latin America.

iatro gave further terms named iatrogenic – harms as a result of medical therapy.

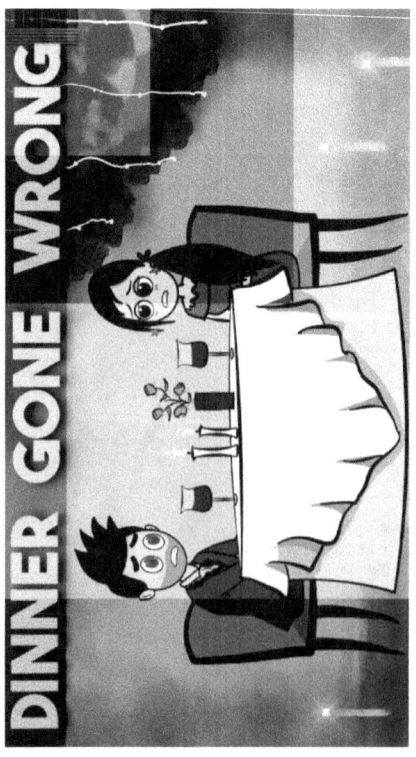

Jatropha is popular folk medicine to relieve bellyache, by causing purging action, thus its fruit is known as bellyache nut.

AS I AM PHYSICIAN'S NUT TO AMPLY BY RECTAL SPHINCTER LAX

Jatropha is popular folk medicine to relieve colicky bellyache, by causing purging action, thus its fruit is known as physician's nut or physic nut.

CANDLE LIGHT DINNER: TOXIC RIDDLE FOR THE TOXIC DETECTIVE

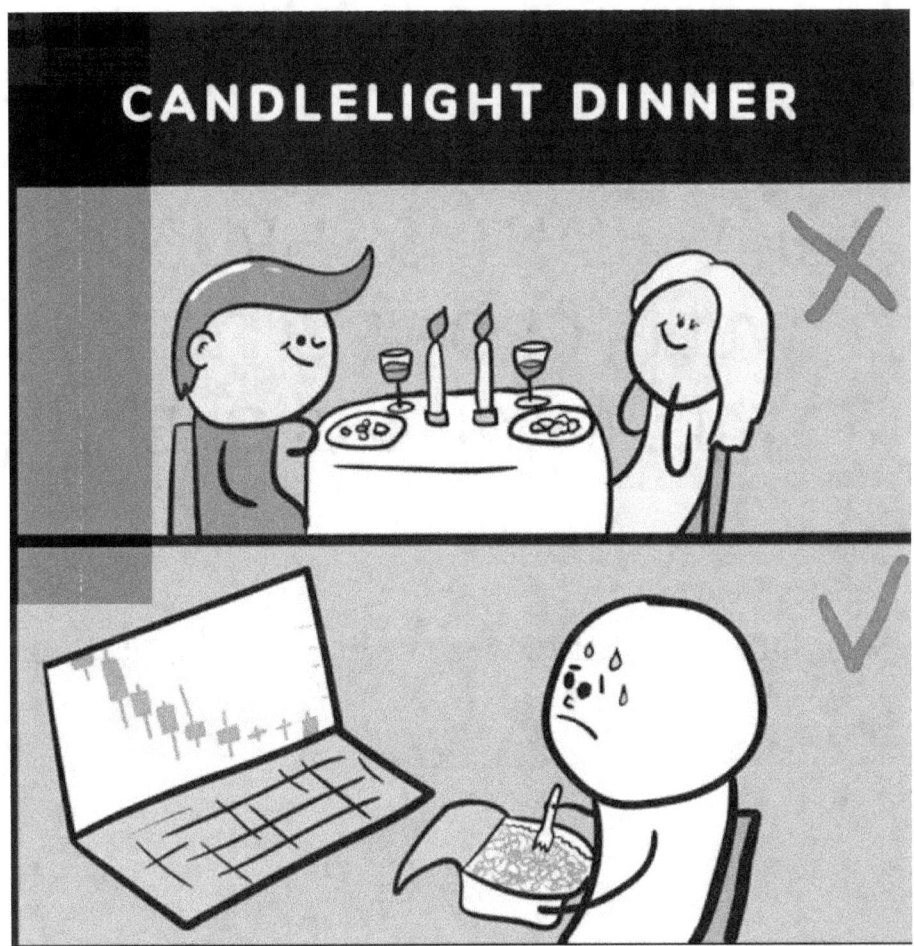

MY PLANT IS SHRUB-WEED, GROWS 5-FEET TALL IN WILD BLOKE;

Tolerates average to poor soils.

Tolerates drought.

Plants will self-seed and have the potential to spread, thus classified as unwanted weed.

I RELIEVE YOUR HURTING BELLYACHE, BUSH THUS MAKE YOU RELAX

Bellyache Bush is another name of Jatropha

HANDS PROTECTING LAMPS

Hope you remember, we use our both hands to protect candle flame from winds in stormy night blowing away the light, when electricity is gone.

PALMATE LEAVES HAVE 5 LOBES, LIKE 5 FINGERS IN UR HANDS □ SEEN;

Maple-like, 3-5 lobed, pale green leaves (to 5" wide) are cordate at the bases.

All 5's for easy recall.

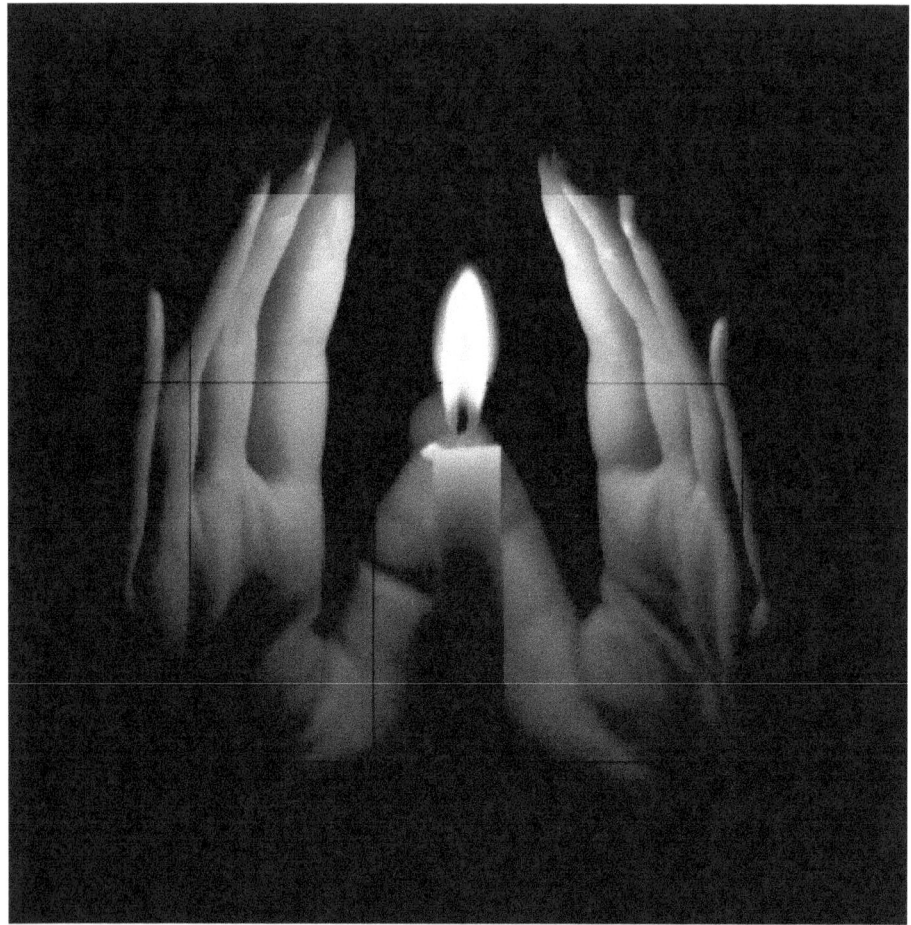

Figure 1. Hands protecting Lamps

Its leaves are like the hands with five fingers, which are grown to fence & protect the delicate & useful plants, just like we in our childhood, used our hands, to save the burning lamp from strong winds.

CANDLE LIGHT DINNER: TOXIC RIDDLE FOR THE TOXIC DETECTIVE

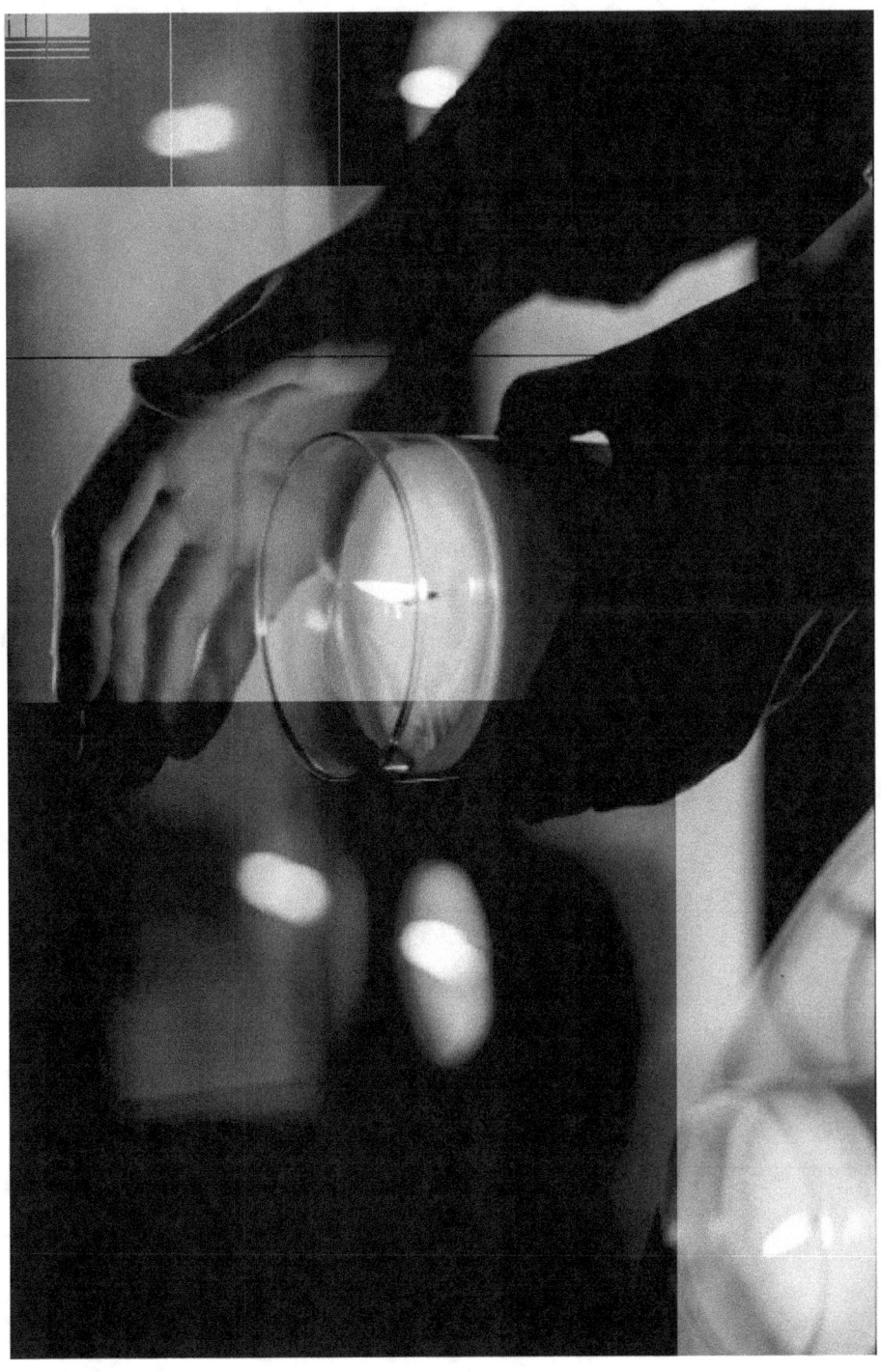

Figure 2. Hands protecting Lamps

Lamps are of wax, made from oil of Jatropha, thus Jatropha is not only the fuel generator for tractors in field, but also the crop protector, as the live fence.

MY BEAN-LIKE SEEDS LOOK-ALIKE BEETLE BLACKENED WITH 5-SPOKE;

Seeds of Jatropha are black in colour & oval alike beetles with back having vertical grroves

ROUTES OF ENTRY: Oral

All cases of systemic poisoning have resulted from ingestion of plant material (in most cases the seeds).

Absorption by route of exposure

INGESTION: Phytotoxins are well absorbed from the gastrointestinal tract.

The onset of symptoms may be developed one or more hours (>50minutes- another 5 for easy recall).

I AM POPULAR, AS FOLK-REMEDIES FOR ABORTING ILLEGALLY IN TEEN;

Jatropha is popular Abortifacient in folk remedies.

Goonasekera MM, Gunawardana VK, Jayasena K, Mohammed SG, Balasubramaniam S. Pregnancy terminating effect of Jatropha curcas in rats. J Ethnopharmacol. 1995 Jul 28;47(3):117-23. doi: 10.1016/0378-8741(95)01263-d. PMID: 8569234.

I AM GROWN FOR INDUSTRIAL BIODIESEL USE IN LANDSCAPING CLOAK;

Jatropha curcas, commonly called purging nut, Barbados nut or physic nut, is a dioecious small tree or large shrub that grows native to Central America, Mexico and the Caribbean, but has been widely planted throughout the tropics for a number of commercial uses, perhaps now most predominately for production of biofuel.

SO CHERRIES REMOVED BY PLANTATIONS BEFORE THEY MATURE IN,

Since its fruits contain seeds, and sweet in taste, so its known as cherries.

As main toxicity & oil is from the fruit seeds, so it is removed from the Jatropha plants, by its farmers, before the fruit ripens, to prevent accidental toxicity among playing kids & grazing animals of his household.

HIGH RISK CIRCUMSTANCES

As these plants are grown as an ornamental they will often be found in gardens and public areas and therefore will be easily accessible.

As Jatropha are fruit bearing and the seeds have a pleasant taste, the plants are particularly attractive to children.

This species of plant is not usually eaten by animals but drought leading to an acute shortage of grass creates a situation in which animals are forced to consume the plants and their constituents in varying amounts.

Citation: http://www.inchem.org/documents/pims/plant/jcurc.htm

OIL-RICH SEEDS CONTAIN, TOXIN KNOWN TO BY SEIZURE & CHOKE,

Its toxin causes cholinergic toxidrome, causing profuse secretions in airway, hypoxia & associated drowsiness & seizures

LEAVES HAVE TOOTHED SERRATED MARGINS GROWING AS WEED, BEEN

Leaves are serrated, just like barbed wire warning to not touch or play with it, s its poisonous. So its considered as weed, and not grown commercially in past.

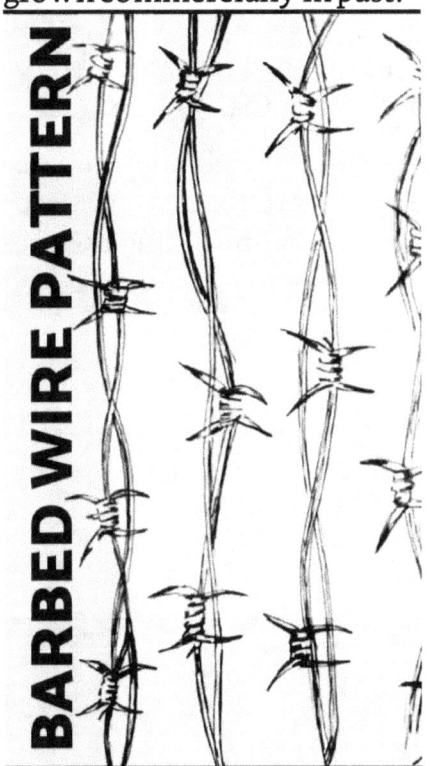

BARBED WIRE PATTERN

BARB 'A' DOSE NUTS IN FRUIT, 3-SEEDED CAPSULE SEEMS TO CONVOKE

Barb-A-dose = Barbados (homophonic) sound alike

Dose means a medication given in measured amount to relieve the suffering patient.

Since Jatropha relieved bellyache in a single dose, and it's also used as barb wire, to protect the fields of farming.

Barbed wire fence are used now, instead of toxic plants, but barb-A-dose Nuts name might have originated for toxic Jatropha's economic purpose just like a barb wire fence, in protecting the precious crop from grazing animals.

CANDLE LIGHT DINNER: TOXIC RIDDLE FOR THE TOXIC DETECTIVE

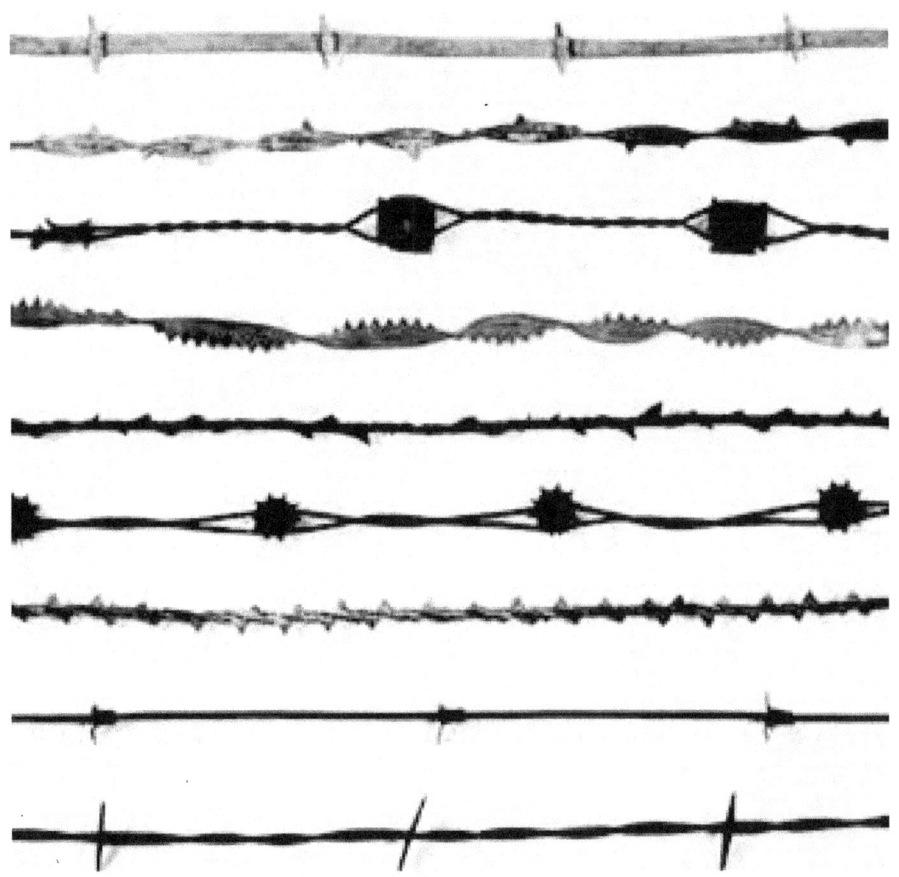

Barbed wire fence for crops
Barb-A-dose= barbados Nut

I AM USED IN MAKING THE PESTICIDES, VARNISHES, SYNTHETIC RESINS

This genera also may contain hydrocyanic acid (CRC Critical Reviews in Toxicology 1977).

There may be a dermatitis producing resin (Lampe & Fagerstrom, 1968).

There may be an alkaloid, and a glycoside which produce cardiovascular and respiratory depression.

Tetramethylpyrazine (TMPZ), an amide alkaloid hasbeen obtained from the stem of J. podagrica (Ojewole & Odebiyi, 1981).

Atropine-like effects have also been reported following ingestion of Jatropha multifida (Aplin 1976).

AS NETTLE SPURGES, USE 5 PERSONAL PROTECTIVE EQUIPMENTS, FOLKS

GLOVES, MASKs, GOWNS , SHOES & GOGGLES, AS PROTECTIVE SHIELDS

Contains a purgative oil and a phytotoxin or toxalbumin (curcin) similar to ricin in Ricinis.

Since Jatropha is irritant to skin and causes cytotoxicity & carcinogenic, so its treated as hazardous substance, just like cytotoxic anticancer agents, and PPE is necessary while handling this plant related toxicity to prevent secondary exposure among healthcare workers.

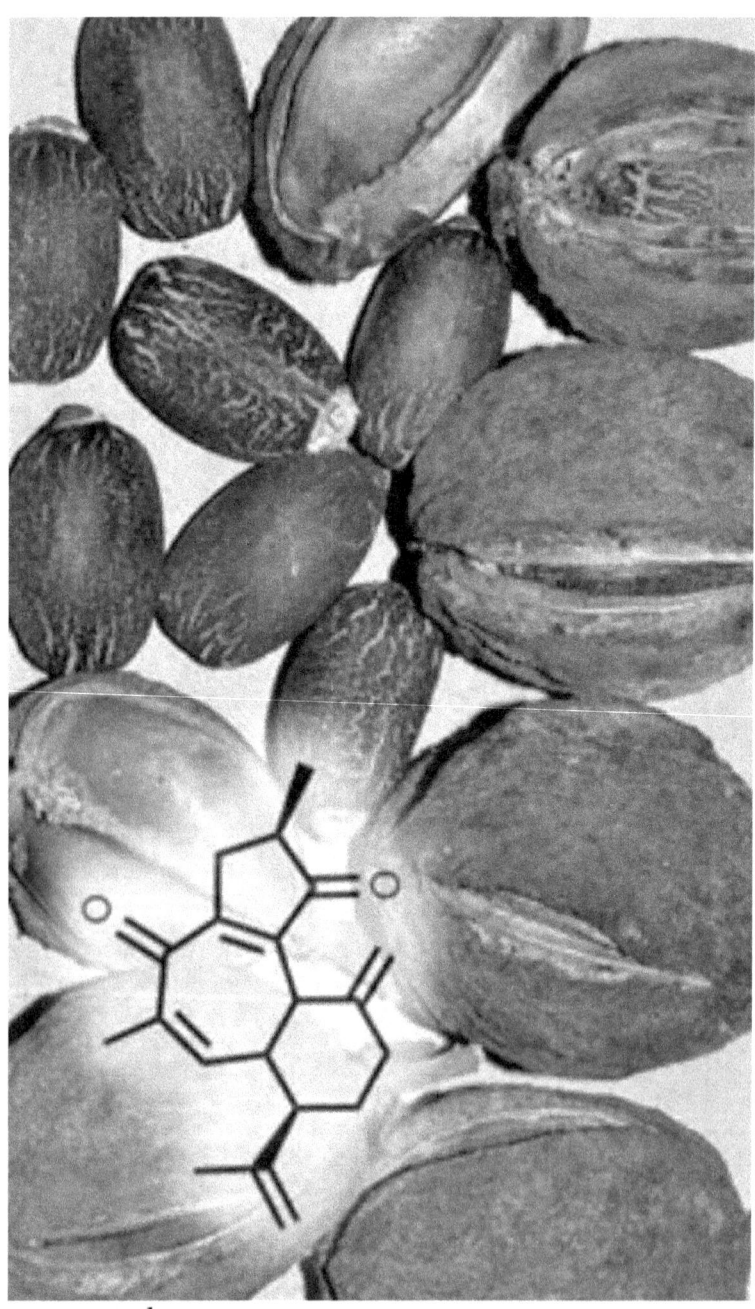

Jatropha curcas = Ratan-Jyot, having Phorbol toxin

AS MY OIL OF POISON NUT & RIPE FRUIT, LOOK YELLOW ALIKE EGG YOLKS

Ripe fruit is yellow in colour, and the size of poultry bird's egg

Oil extracted is yellow in colour like egg yolk.

Waxes burn with a yellow flame due to the presence of carbon.

If gastric lavage is done of Jatropha intoxicated victims within an hour, than thick yellowish viscid gastric aspirate is diagnostic clue.

SO MY PLANTS WERE USED AS LIVE FENCES TO GUARD YOUR GRAIN FIELDS

It is cultivated in almost all tropical and subtropical countries as protection hedges around gardens and fields, since it is not browsed by cattle.

Barbed wire are used now, instead of toxic plants, but barb-A-dose Nuts name might have originated for toxic Jatropha's economic purpose just like a barb wire fence, in protecting the precious crop from grazing animals.

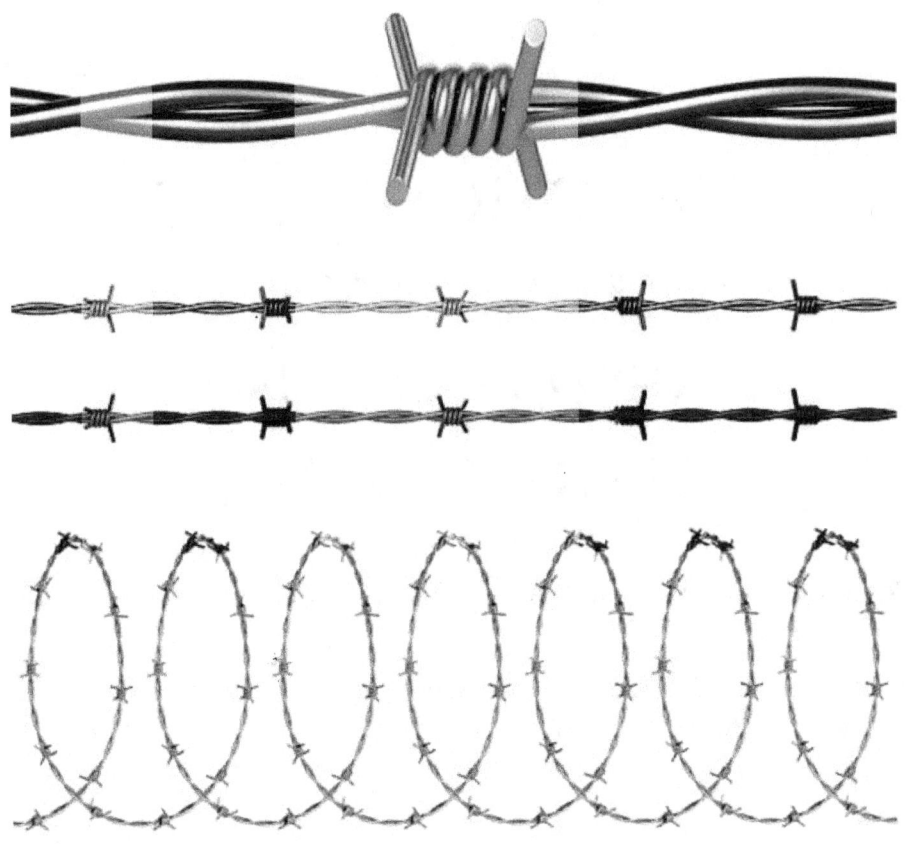

Barb Wire Fence Barbed Wire
Barb-A-dose= Barbados (homophonic) sound alike, its nature's defence to Jatropha, from its herbivore predators, as its fruit & seeds are sweet & palatable to eat, but irritant & toxic on ingestion

THE TOXIC DOSE TO SICKEN ANIMALS TRESPASSING IS 5 SEEDS TO POKE

Poisonous parts: All parts are considered toxic but in particular the seeds.

Main toxins: Contains a purgative oil and a phytotoxin or toxalbumin (curcin) similar to ricin in Ricinis.

DITERPENOIDS OF TIGLIANE & PHORBOL ARE CARCINOGENIC INTO YIELDS

Phorbol is carcinogenic

Phorbol esters are the tetracyclic diterpenoids generally known for their tumor promoting activity.

The phorbol esters mimic the action of diacyl glycerol (DAG), activator of protein kinase C, which regulates different signal transduction pathways and other cellular metabolic activities.

They occur naturally in many plants of the family Euphorbiacaeae and Thymelaeaceae.

The biological activities of the phorbol esters are highly structure specific.

The phorbol esters, even at very low concentrations, show toxicological manifestations in animals fed diets containing them.

This toxicity limits the use of many nutritive plants and agricultural by-products containing phorbol esters to be used as animal feed.

Therefore, various chemical and physical treatments have been evaluated to extract or inactivate phorbol esters so that seed meals rich in proteins could be used as feed resources.

However, not much progress has been reported so far.

The detoxifying ability has also been reported in some molluscs and in liver homogenate of mice.

Besides, possessing antinutritional and toxic effects, few derivatives of the phorbol esters are also known for their antimicrobial and antitumor activities.

The molluscicidal and insecticidal properties of phorbol esters indicate its potential to be used as an effective biopesticide and insecticide.

Goel G, Makkar HP, Francis G, Becker K. Phorbol esters: structure, biological activity, and toxicity in animals. Int J Toxicol. 2007 Jul-Aug;26(4):279-88. doi: 10.1080/10915810701464641. PMID: 17661218.

COAGULANT & ANTICOAGULANT ACTIVITIES IN JATROPHA CURCAS LATEX

Jatropha curcas Linn. (Euphorbiaceae), a medicinal plant commonly grown in the Tropics, is traditionally used as a haemostatic.

IN LOWER CONCENTRATE, I'M ANTICOAGULANT CURE STROKE

Investigation by Omolaja O., ey al. (2003) at Department of Biochemistry, Obafemi Awolowo University, Ile-Ife 22005, Nigeria, of the coagulant activity of the latex of Jatropha curcas showed that whole latex significantly reduced the clotting time of human blood.

I'M EXPERIMENTAL HEMOSTATIC AGENT, IF BLEED SOAKS

Diluted latex, however, prolonged the clotting time: at high dilutions, the blood did not clot at all.

This indicates that Jatropha curcas latex possesses both procoagulant and anticoagulant activities.

Prothrombin time (PT) and activated partial thromboplastin time (APTT) tests on plasma confirm these observations.

Solvent partitioning of the latex with ethyl acetate and butanol led to a partial separation of the two opposing activities: at low concentrations, the ethyl acetate fraction exhibited a procoagulant activity, while the butanol fraction had the highest anticoagulant activity

Omolaja O., ey al. Coagulant and anticoagulant activities in Jatropha curcas latex. Journal of Ethnopharmacology 89 (2003) 101–105.

BY GENETIC ENGINEERING, MY NON-TOXIC VARIETY CULTURED IN SEEDS

Single nucleotide polymorphism diversity in non-toxic jatropha is relatively high, particularly in northern Veracruz state, the probable origin of this germplasm.

Genetic differences between toxic and non-toxic indigenous genotypes are overall quite small.

A genome-wide association study supported a genomic region (on LG 8, scaffold NW_012130064), probably involved in the suppression of seed toxicity.

Conservation actions are urgently needed to preserve this non-toxic indigenous, relatively wild germplasm, having potential as a fuel feedstock, animal feed and food source among other uses.

More generally, this work demonstrates the value of conservation genomic research on the indigenous gene pool of economically important plant species.

Vandepitte K, et al. High SNP diversity in the non-toxic indigenous Jatropha curcas germplasm widens the potential of this upcoming major biofuel crop species. Ann Bot. 2019 Oct 29;124(4):645-652. doi: 10.1093/aob/mcz008. PMID: 30715120;

PMCID: PMC6821362.

I'M MULTIPURPOSE HERBAL GOLDMINE, TO ENRICH IN OILY BEAN SOAKS

Jatropha curcas (jatropha) is an oil crop cultivated in (sub)tropical regions around the world, and holds great promise as a renewable energy source for biodiesel.

MY STEM BARK OR LATEX IS USED FOR HUNTING FISH POISON TO NEEDS

The Jatropha bark was being as a fish poison for hunting fishes by tribals in Africa.

JATROPHA

Jatropha is a genus of flowering plants in the spurge family, Euphorbiaceae, belongs to tribe Joanneasiae of Crotonoideae in the Euphorbiaceae family and contains approximately 175 species, cultivated throughout the tropical to temperate regions of the world.

Family: Euphorbiaceae

- ➢ Jatropha cathartica Terán & Berland.
- ➢ Jatropha curcas L.
- ➢ Jatropha gossypifolia L.
- ➢ Jatropha integerrima Jacq. and varieties
- ➢ Jatropha macrorhiza Benth.
- ➢ Jatropha multifida L.
- ➢ Jatropha podagrica Hook.

The name is derived from the Greek words ἰατρός (iatros), meaning "physician", and τροφή (trophe), meaning "nutrition", hence the common name physic nut.

Another common name is nettlespurge

Common names in English include physic nut, Barbados nut, poison nut, bubble bush or purging nut

Jatropha curcas L. and J. macrocarpa Griseb: Seed Morphology, Viability, Dormancy, Germination and Growth of Seedlings. Au-

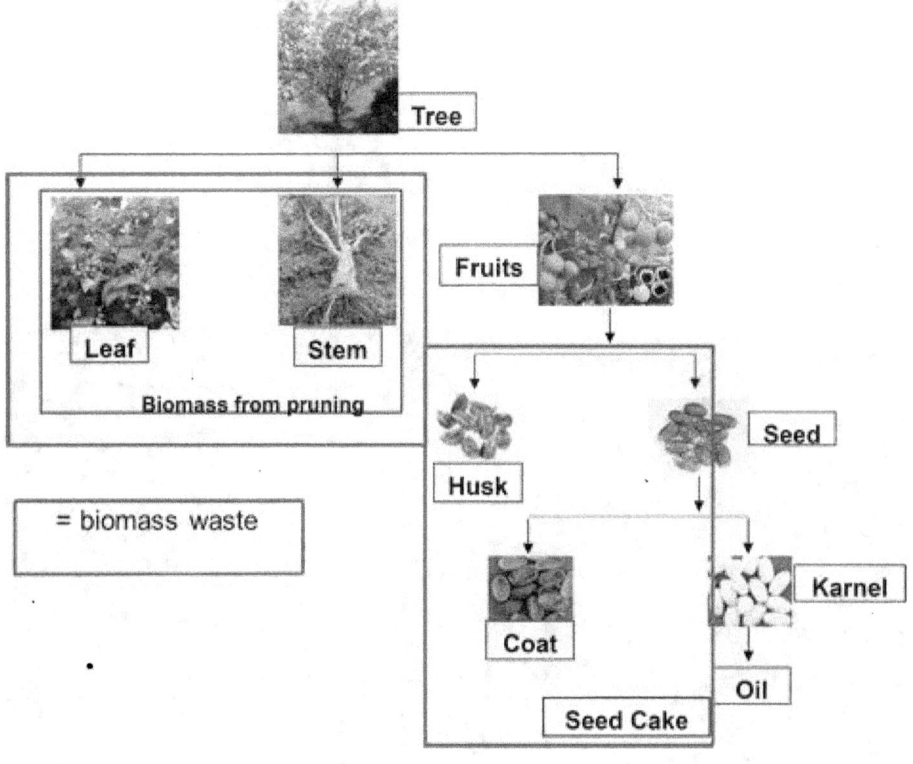

CLASSIFICATION

Cell toxin, co-carcinogen, skin irritant; highly hazardous (Ib).

TM: Central and South America, Europe (now obsolete).

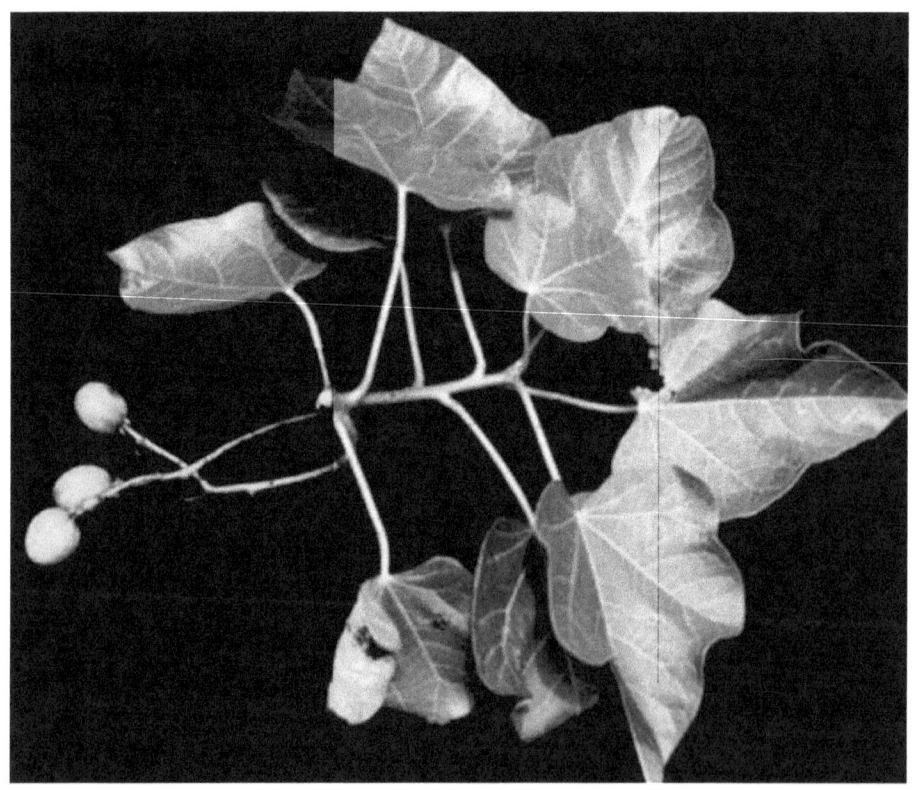

USES & PROPERTIES

Its seeds are rich in oil (ca. 35%) that was once used as a purgative medicine to treat constipation.

Jatropha species have traditionally been used in basketmaking, tanning and dye production.

In the 2000s, one species, Jatropha curcas, generated interest as an oil crop for biodiesel production and also medicinal importance when used as lamp oil.

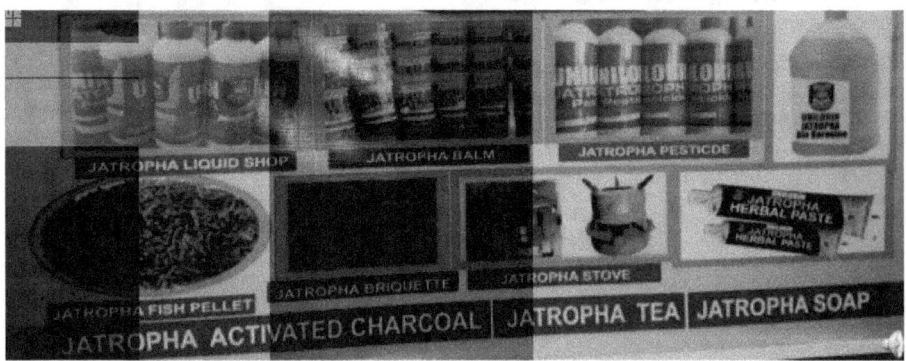

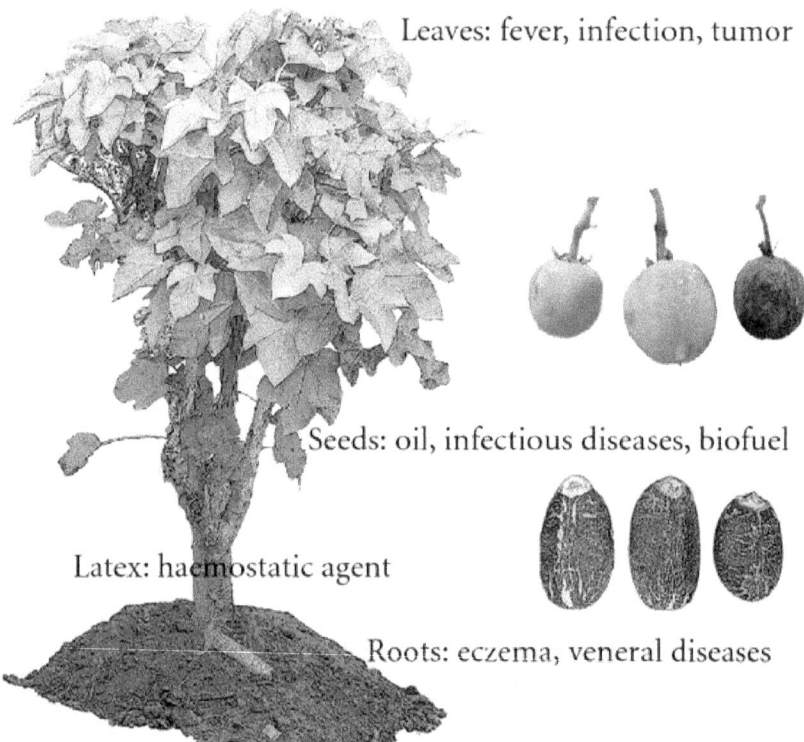

ORIGIN

Tropical America. Grown in Central America, India and Africa as live fences and nowadays on a commercial scale for biofuel production.

SPECIAL IDENTIFICATION FEATURES

Jatropha curcas is a large coarse annual shrub 5 feet height or small short lived tree which can grow 5 meters tall.

It has thin, often greenish bark which exudes copious amounts of watery sap when cut.

Leaves: dark green; alternate, simple, ovate to slightly lobed with 3-5 indentations.

Leaves are Up to 5 inches wide.

Petioles (the stalk that joins a leaf to a stem) is 4-5 inches long.

Flowers: yellow to green in colour, borne in axils of the leaves and being small are mostly hidden by foliage.

Fruit: small capsule-like, round fruit; about 2.5 - 5cm in diameter.

These are green and fleshy when immature, becoming dark brown when ripe and splitting to release 2 or 3 black seeds each about 2 cm (3/4 inch) long.

The meat of the seeds is white, and oily in texture and are reported to have an agreeable taste.

3D'S MNEMONIC

- D-Diarrhoea
- D-Dehydration
- D-Delirium

CASTOR VS JATROPHA

- Both have all 5's to easy recall
- Both seeds are toxic
- Both produces oil for economic use as biofuel
- Jatropha is aka jungli arandi, as it's a weed like castor (arandi) एरण्डतैल, found in forests (jungle), and produces oil from seeds

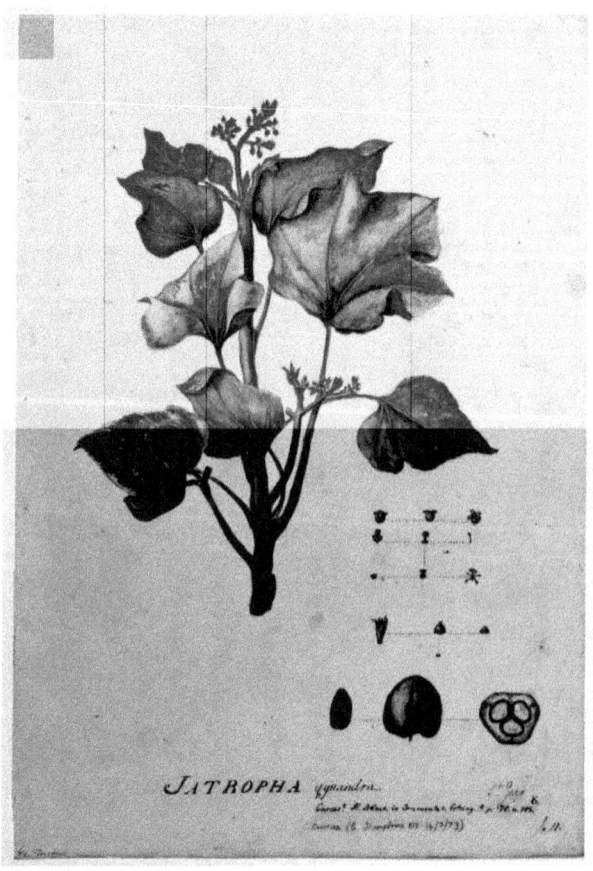

CHEMISTRY

MY PLANT HAS CURE QUEUE SON AC COOL TO WIND BROKE;

CURE -QUEUE- SON= cur-cu-sone =curcusone (homophonic)

AC= A and C.

Diterpenoids of the tigliane (phorbol) type, mainly curcusone A and C.

AC stands for Air Conditioner, providing cool breeze of wind.

Jatropha plants were planted on fences of the farms as Wind Breakers, to prevent the strong winds to take away the fertile humus from the farm fields, just when the seeds of commercial plants are sown.

Thus Jatropha as a large shrub in row was used in arid zones, where desert storms are common, to maintain the fertility of soil.

Seed contains a very poisonous lectin (toxic protein/ toxalbumin) known as curcin or jatrophin.

It is absent from oil (not fat-soluble).

Phytotoxins are heat labile, and can be positively identified by precipitin reactions with sera containing known antibodies (Kingsbury 1964).

Curcanoleic acid is present in the oil

(cf. ricinoleic acid in castor oil).

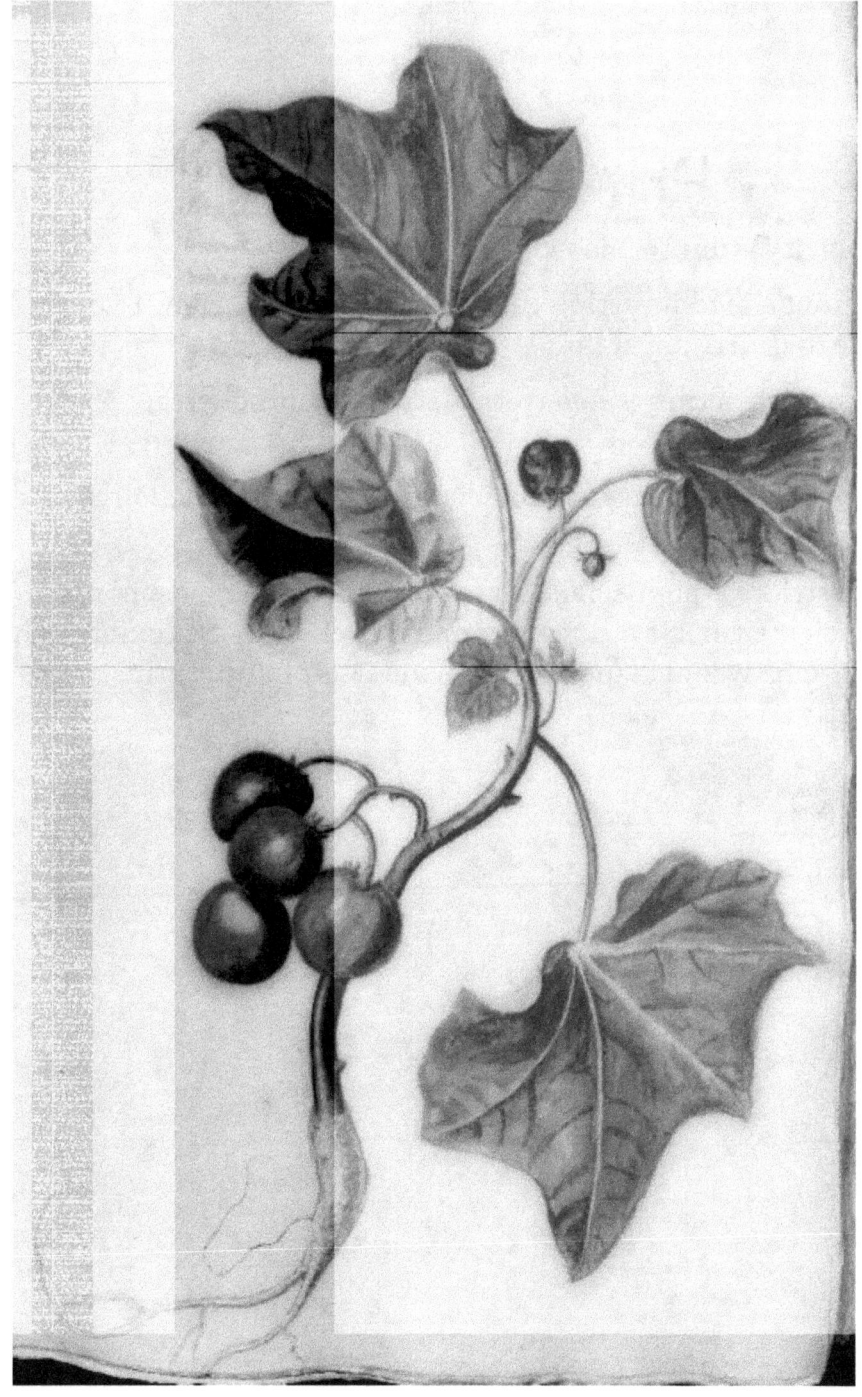

PHARMACOLOGY

Toxicity is due to phorbol esters and curcin.

Jatropha seed ingestion causes diarrhoea, delirium & vomiting, due to its irritant action.

Purgative action is due to the irritant phorbol esters & curcanoleic acid.

Hypersalivation, sweating & polyuria, due acetylcholine receptor stimulation is noted.

Constricted pupils raises a doubt of organophosphorus (OP) pesticide toxicity, since it simulates cholinergic toxicity, thus Jatropha was also used as pesticide itself in rural tribal areas in past.

USES

Jatropha is an ornamental plant naturalised in many tropical areas.

The roots, stems, leaves seeds and fruits of the plant have been widely used in traditional folk medicine in many parts of Africa & India.

The seeds of J. curcas have been used as a purgative, antihelminthic and abortifacient as well as for treating ascites, gout, paralysis and skin diseases.

The seed oil of the plant has been used as an ingredient in the treatment of rheumatic conditions, itch and parasitic skin diseases, and in the treatment of fever, jaundice and gonorrhoea, as a diuretic agent, and a mouth-wash.

The leaf has been used as a haemostatic agent and the bark as a fish poison.

In certain African countries people are accustomed to chewing these seeds when in need of a laxative.

HOMEOPATHIC USES

Homeopathically it is used for cold sweats, colic, cyanosis, and leg cramps.

Viswanathan, MBG, et al. Review on Jatropha. International Journal of Research and Innovation in Social Science (IJRISS) |Volume II, Issue VIII, August 2018

ANTIHELMINTHIC

J. curcas seeds have been found to be highly effective against Strongyloides papillosus infection in goats (Adam & Magzoub, in press).

It has also been suggested that J. curcas seeds could be a useful chemotherapeutic agent provided that it is active at a non-lethal dose (Adam, 1974).

This may be because of it's reported antihelminthic activity.

ANTICANCER CYTOTOXIC

Recently Zhang Y., et al., in 2017 identified a novel type I ribosome-inactivating protein (RIP), designated as curcin C, was purified from Jatropha curcas, an important feedback source of biofuel.

It exhibited N-glycosidase activity and in vitro translation inhibition activity.

Moreover, curcin C displayed a strong selectively anti-tumor activity on human cancer cells.

Its cytotoxicity against osteosarcoma cell line U2OS is even higher than that of Paclitaxel with IC50 of 0.019 μM.

Purification and identification of curcin C not only suggested its potential in natural anticancer drug development, but also provide chance to understanding different cytotoxic action among different RIPs.

Zhang Y., et al., Curcin C, a novel type I ribosome-inactivating protein from the post-germinating cotyledons of Jatropha curcas. Amino Acids. 2017 Sep;49(9):1619-1631.

Phorbol is a natural, plant-derived organic compound. It is a member of the tigliane family of diterpenes. Phorbol was first isolated in 1934 as the hydrolysis product of croton oil, which is derived from the seeds of the purging croton, Croton tiglium

JATROPHA CURCAS LEAVES ON TURTLE HEART

Estrada, , Horacio, R , Quintin L. Kintanar, , Trinidad, JT , Ambay, B . "Effect of Jatropha curcas leaves on turtle heart preparation" Acta Med Philipp (2): 60-61, 1974

ANTI-ARRHYTHMIC

Preliminary pharmacological studies by Fojas, et al. (1986) of Jatropha curcas (JC) or "tubang bakod" leaves suggest that this plant has potent cardiovascular action and is a possible source of an anti-arrhythmic (beta blocker) agent.

Experiments on guinea pig showed decreased heart force (negative inotropic), decreased heart rate (negative chronotropic) and blocking of the isoprenaline stimulation responses on the auricle which is somewhat similar to a well-known beta-blocker, propranolol.

Other findings indicate that the plant is a central depressant with some sympathomimetic activity and a potent drug with LD50 values of: 24.5 g/kg (18.15 g/kg - 33.08 g/kg) and 750 mg/kg (517 mg/kg - 1087 mg/kg), for the aqueous extract (decoction) and methanol extract, respectively.

Fojas. F.R., Garia, L.L., Venzon, E.L., Sison, F.M.,Villamiera, B.A., Jojas, A.J. and Liava, I. (1986). Pharmaceutical studies of Jatropha curcas as a possible source of anti-arrhythmic (beta blocker) agent. Phillippine Journal of Science, 115: 317-328.

TOXICOLOGY

As with many members of the family Euphorbiaceae, Jatropha contains compounds that are highly toxic.

Lethal when injected but relatively low oral toxicity: 5 to 20 seeds cause toxic effects.

Curcin: Phytotoxins or toxalbumins are large, complex protein molecules of high toxicity.

They resemble bacterial toxins in structure and physiological effects.

Curcin is said to be highly irritant and remains in the seed after the oil has been expressed.

Tetramethylpyrazine (TMPZ):
- CAS: 1124-11-4
- MW: 136.22
- Molecular formula: C8-H12-N2

Much like other members of the family Euphorbiaceae, members of the genus Jatropha contain several toxic compounds.

The seeds of Jatropha curcas contain the highly poisonous toxalbumin curcin, a lectin dimer.

They also contain carcinogenic phorbol.

LETHAL DOSE

The LD50 of the ethanol extract of the Jatropha Cucas (JC) seed was determined by the method initially described by Lorke (1983).

In addition, acute behavioral and CNS toxicity studies of JC including antidotal therapy against JC poisoning were done.

The LD50 of IP JC extract ranged from 177.48 to 288.53 mg/kg (moderately toxic) for the adult female rat, adult male mouse and young male rat.

For the adult male rats the LD50 values were 565.69 mg/kg (IP, slightly toxic) and >5000 mg/kg (oral, slightly toxic) and the LD50 of the JC extract for the chicks was 28.28 mg/kg (IP, highly toxic).

Citation: Lorke, D. (1983). A new approach to practical acute toxicity testing. Arch Toxicol, 54: 275-287.

ANTIDOTES

JC produced a fairly dose dependent behavioral and CNS depressant effects which were reduced by atropine, EDTA and a combination of atropine, sodium nitrite & sodium thiosulphate, and EDTA.

Also these antidotes either singly or in combination reduced mortality among the rats by 25-50%.

Citation: Abiri, OT., et al, Acute toxicity studies and antidotal therapy of ethanol extract of jatropha curcas seeds in experimental animals. Sierra Leone J Biomed Res Dec. 2015, Vol 7, No 2.

DIAGNOSIS

Toxidromic Diagnosis is made by case history & presenting symptoms.

A definite diagnosis can only be made if there is a history of ingestion and the ingested plant material has been positively identified as Jatropha by physical findings & chemical analysis.

VOMITING, DELIRIUM, DIARRHEA ARE COMMON SYMPTOMS, U SPOKE

Main risks & target organs:

Dehydration and cardiovascular collapse are, as a result of haemorrhagic gastro-enteritis.

Symptoms are largely those associated with gastro-intestinal irritation.

There is acute abdominal pain and a burning sensation in the throat about half an hour after ingestion of the seeds, followed by nausea, vomiting and diarrhoea.

The vomitus and faeces may contain blood.

In severe intoxications dehydration and haemorrhagic gastro-enteritis can occur.

There may be CNS and cardiovascular depression and collapse; children are more susceptible.

FIRST-AID MEASURES

INGESTION: Unless the patient is unconscious, convulsing, or unable to swallow give fluids (milk or water) to dilute. Seek medical assistance.

In hospital or a health care facility induce stomach wash, unless the patient has already vomited, and perform gastric lavage. Administer activated charcoal to adsorb the phytotoxin, Whole Bowel irrigation by PEGLAC for cathartic action may hasten elimination, although in the presence of diarrhoea, this is unnecessary.

SKIN: Wash the affected area well with plenty of water and use a mild soap.

EYE: Flush the eye with copious amounts of water for at least 15 minutes. If irritation persists seek medical assistance.

ILLUSTRATIVE CASES OF JATROPHA POISONING

Case reports from literature

I'M KNOWN TO CAUSE BLACK VOMIT, NUT IF THE VICTIM ANIMAL FEEDS

Black vomit nut is another name of Jatropha curcas.

Blackish vomitus is due to black coloured seed coatings of Jatropha plant, which are easily chewable, but irritant to gastrointestinal tract.

CASE HISTORY 1: JATROPHA CURCAS SEEDS

Ho RKB., et al in 1960 reported that a 3-year-old Hawaiian-Caucasian boy was admitted to Kauikeoani Children's Hospital on September 20, 1958, because of persistent vomiting and diarrhoea.

The episodes were of sudden onset following the ingestion of several large black seeds gathered from an over-hanging branch of a neighbour's tree (later identified as Jatropha curcas).

He was unable to retain any ingested food or water.

Each intake was vomited almost immediately after ingestion.

The vomitus was said to contain the white granulated material and the particles of the black shells.

After several bouts of vomiting, the child started to have watery bowel movements.

The stools contained seed particles also.

Three and a half hours following the ingestion of the seeds, the child appeared lethargic.

His skin felt cold and clammy.

The child was admitted to the hospital in severe dehydration.

The family and past history were non-contributory.
Blood pressure was 100/70; pulse 130; respiration 40; temperature 99.8°F (rectal).
The patient appeared lethargic, cyanotic, and acutely ill.
The peripheral vessels were constricted.
Severe dehydration was indicated by the poor skin turgor, sunken eyeballs, and deepening periorbital shadows.
The bowel sounds were hyperactive.
The remainder of the physical examination was within normal limits.

The haemoglobin was 14.2gm/100mL, the red blood cell count, 5.4 million, and the platelets were normal.

The white blood cell count was 27,000 per cu mm, and the differential was normal.

The urine showed a trace of albumin, and elements consisting of 2-4 white blood cells per high power field and many granular and some hyaline casts.

The carbon oxide level was 17mEq/L; chlorides, 101mEq/L; and potassium, 4.4mEq/L.

The stool cultures were negative for pathogens.

The child was given 1000mL of isotonic electrolyte solution.

Blood was drawn for type and cross matching.

The patient was oliguric for the first 24 hours.

He responded to treatment, and twenty hours after admission he was able to tolerate oral feedings without any vomiting or diarrhoea, and was voiding well.

He was discharged from the hospital after 3 days without complication.

Citation: Ho Richard K B. (March-April 1960). Acute Poisoning From the Ingestion of Seeds of Jatropha Curcas. Medical Journal of Hawaii, 19(4):421-423.

CASE HISTORY 2: J. CURCAS SEEDS

Abdu-Aguye et al., in 1986 reported that two sisters aged 5 and 3 years respectively were rushed to Ahmadu Bello University Teaching Hospital, Zaria, Nigeria, with a history of vomiting and drowsiness about 5 hours after ingesting unspecified quantities of ripe seeds of J. curcas.

They had each vomited between 6 and 10 times within the hour preceding their arrival.

There had been no diarrhea and the vomitus consisted of a whitish material mixed with the food they had taken 2 hour previously.

On examination they were well-fed children, afebrile, not pale, jaundiced or cyanosed but moderately dehydrated.
There was neither abdominal tenderness nor any abnormal finding on rectal examination.
They were restless, drowsy but arousable and their pupils were normal and reactive. Laboratory investigations revealed normal haemoglobin, normal liver-function tests and mild alkalosis.

Treatment consisted of rehydration with intravenous fluids and sedation with small doses of promethazine hydrochloride.

They recovered rapidly and were both discharged some 48 hours after admission.

Citation: Abdu-Aguye I, A Sannusi, R A Alafiya-Tayo, S R Bhusnurmath. (Jul 1986) Acute Toxcity Studies with Jatropha curcas L. Human Toxicology, 5(4):269-274.

CASE SERIES 1: JATROPHA CURCAS SEEDS, FOOD POISONING AS ENDEMIC IN AFRICAN KIDS

During the first 3 months of 1983, 8 children were admitted to Ga-Aankuwa Hospital with marked nausea, vomiting and diarrhoea after ingesting the seeds of Jatropha curcas.

Joubert, et al., in 1984 reported that these poisonings occurred in children between the ages of 2 and 9 years (4 male, 4 female) who thought the seeds were edible.

All presented with moderate to marked gastrointestinal symptoms, including nausea, vomiting and abdominal cramps.

Of these patients, five were clinically dehydrated and were given intravenous fluid replacement.

All patients made a rapid and uneventful recovery and could be discharged the next day.

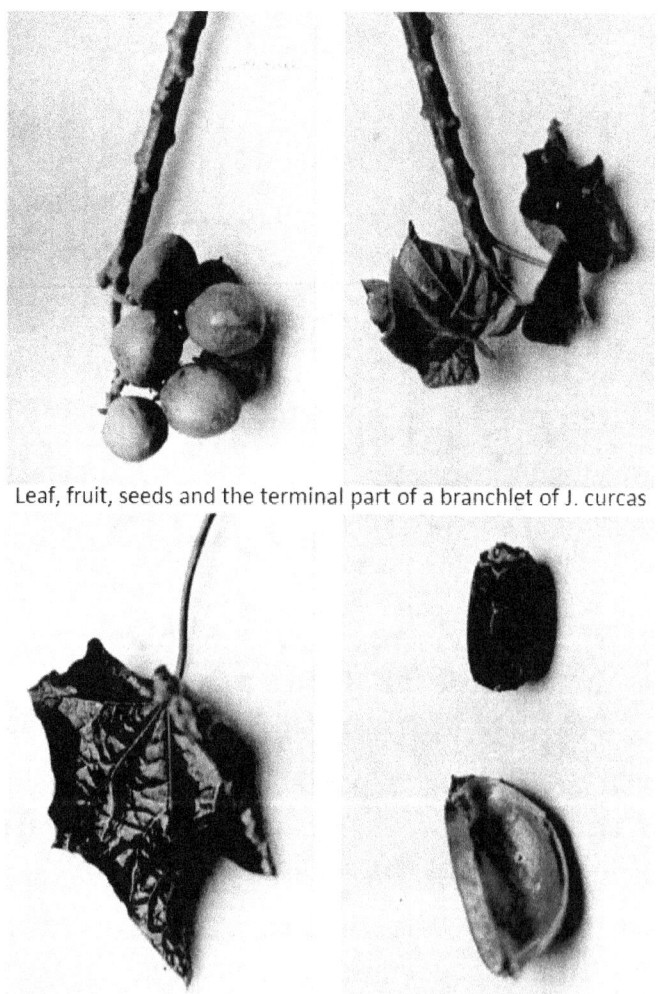

Figure 3. Leaf, fruit, seeds and the terminal part of a branchlet of Jatropha curcas.

Citation: Joubert P H, J M M Brown, I T Hay, P D B Sebata. (May 1984). Acute poisoning with Jatropha curcas (purging nut tree) in children. South African Medical Journal,

65:729-730.

CASE SERIES 2: JATROPHA CURCAS SEEDS, FOOD POISONING IS ENDEMIC IN INDIAN KIDS

From Jan 2004 to Dec 2013, total of 169 cases of Jatropha curcas poisoning were reported by Kosam A., et al. (2014) at Chhattisgarh Institute of Medical Sciences, Bilaspur, Chhattisgarh, India.

Acute Jatropha poisoning was the commonest cause of poisoning in children constituting 31% of poisoning cases.

Vomiting was the most common symptom present in all children followed by abdominal pain (58%), weakness (21%), dehydration (13%) and diarrhea (11%).

Hypovolemia shock was documented in 6 children with acute Jatropha poisoning.

All children required IV fluids, IV anti emetics and ORS. 4 % cases required IV fluid resuscitation & oxygen supplementation due to hypovolemia shock.

Most children who ingest Jatropha curcas seeds develop

mild gastrointestinal symptoms but life threatening complications like hypovolemia shock can occur.

One of the children had constricted pupils raising a doubt of organophosphorus poisoning.

The children denied consuming any liquid chemical.

On further questioning, the children brought out history of consumption of some black coloured seeds which were growing around the school premises.

On examination these seeds were identified to be of Jatropha curcas.

The reasons for ingestion were curiosity and sweet taste of the seeds.

The lag period before onset of symptoms varied between one to two hours.

All the children were given gastric lavage followed by anti-emetics and IV fluids.

Their symptoms subsided within 6-8 hours.

They were observed for 24 hours and discharged the next day.

Health care providers must recognize, assess and initiate appropriate management promptly to minimize the serious consequences that could endanger the lives of the patients.

PREDICTING POISONING DUE TO JATROPHA, COMMONEST IN WINTERS

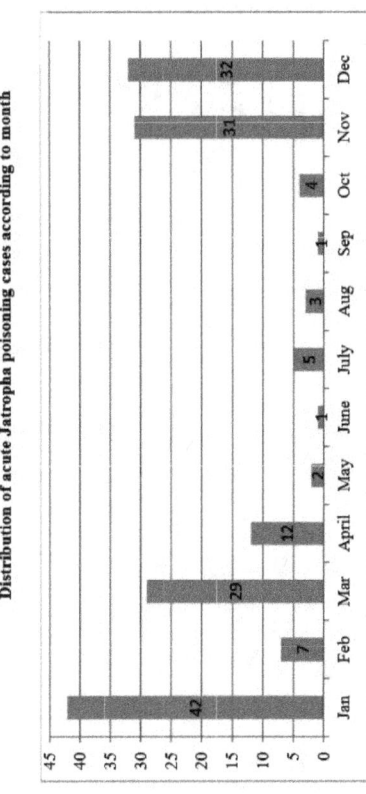

Distribution of acute Jatropha poisoning cases according to month

Figure 4. Predicting poisoning due to Jatropha, commonest in winters. Image source: Kosam A., et al. (2014) Int J Med Res Rev. 2014 Jun.30;2(3):221-7.

Food Poisoning due to accidental consumption of Jatropha seeds is most commonly seen in winters, as fruits occur after flowering season in the winters

Citation:

Kosam A, Nahrel R. Clinical profile of Jatropha Curcas poisoning in children. Int J Med Res Rev. 2014 Jun.30;2(3):221-7.

CASE SERIES 1: JATROPHA MACRORHIZA ROOTS

Consroe and Glow, in 1975 reported that an 18 year old, well developed Caucasian male was admitted to hospital at 11:45 p.m. because of persistent vomiting, diarrhoea and drowsiness.

The patient had ingested 3 pieces (about 2 inches in diameter) of a plant root (identified as Jatropha macrorhiza) about 4 hours earlier; symptoms emerged about 1 hour after ingestion.

Except for drowsiness and tenderness of all quadrants of the abdomen, physical examination and haematologic and urinary laboratory values of the patient showed no striking abnormalities.

Bed rest was prescribed and tap water was given ad libitum to quench the patient's extreme polydipsia.

After an uneventful night's sleep, the patient was discharged at 10:30 the next morning without complications.

Citation: Consroe P F, Glow D E. (1975). Clinical Toxicology of the Desert Potato: Two Case Reports of Acute Jatropha Macrorhiza Root Ingestion. Arizona Medicine, 23(6):475-477.

CONTRARY TO ATROPINE USE, RELIEVE SYMPTOM TO JAY, ATROPINE LEADS

ATROPINE LIKE TOXIDROME WAS REPORTED IN SPECIES MULTIFIDA BROKE

JATROPHA VS ATROPHA

The difference of J, makes its opposite to its toxicity.

CHOLINERGIC TOXIDROME BY JATROPHA: REVERSED BY ANTICHOLINERGIC ATROPHINE

Case series 2: Jatropha macrorhiza roots

Consroe and Glow, in 1975 reported that another case of 48 year old, well developed Caucasian male was admitted to hospital at 3 p.m. because of persistent diarrhoea after ingesting an unknown quantity of a sweet tasting potato-like plant root (identified as Jatropha macrorhiza) at 8 a.m.

Bouts of severe vomiting and diarrhoea about every 3 minutes appeared 45 to 60 minutes after ingestion and persisted throughout most of the afternoon.

The patient also complained of drowsiness, perspiration, salivation, polydipsia, cramps in the legs and abdomen and of feeling cold and clammy.

Physical examination revealed a poor skin turgor, sunken eyeballs excessive salivary secretions and no lesions of mouth or throat.

There was tenderness in all quadrants of the abdomen and deep tendon reflexes were hyperactive and intermittent muscle spasms in toes and calves were apparent.

Vital signs and urinary and haematological values were normal except for elevations in haematocrit (60%) and haemoglobin (20.2gm/100ml).

Initially, 1 litre of 5% dextrose in water, atropine (0.5mg IM.) and diazepam (5mg, IM.) every 6-8 hours as needed were prescribed.

After a restful night, the patient was discharged at 9 a.m., the following morning without complications.

Citation: Consroe P F, Glow D E. (1975). Clinical Toxicology of the Desert Potato: Two Case Reports of Acute Jatropha Macrorhiza Root Ingestion. Arizona Medicine, 23(6):475-477.

http://www.inchem.org/documents/pims/plant/jcurc.htm

AUTOPSY FINDINGS IN JATROPHA TOXICITY

Poisoning by these seeds is well known in forensic practice and autopsy findings include severe gastro-enteritis, nephritis, myocardial degeneration, haemagglutination and subepicardial and subendocardial haemorrhages as well as renal subcortical and subpleural bleeding.

Steyn DG. Vergifciging van Mms m Dier. Pretoria: JL van Schaik, 1949: 151-152.

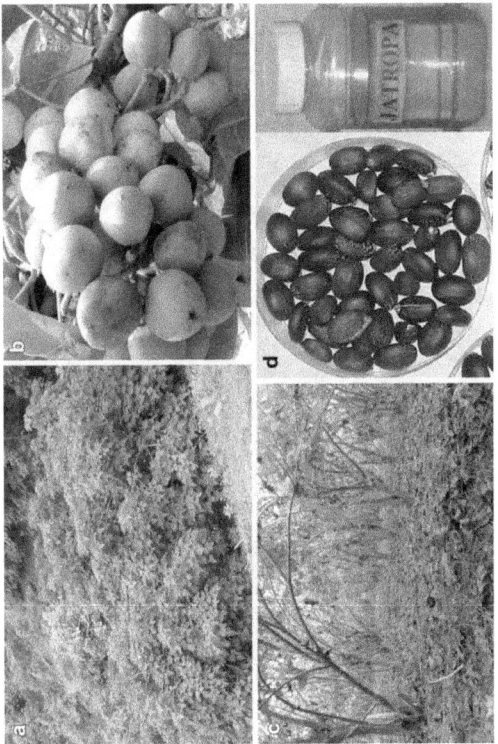

www.ingramcontent.com/pod-product-compliance
Lightning Source LLC
Chambersburg PA
CBHW070423220526
45466CB00004B/1513